The Dash Diet Cookbook

A Natural Solution to Control High Blood Pressure. Cardiovascular Wellness Diet Recipes to Improve Your Health and Live a Disease-Free Life

Ellen Ramsey

TABLE OF CONTENTS

INTRODUCTION

D iet is a very effective diet plan that helps lower blood pressure, and research has shown it is DASH. The nutritional approach to preventing hypertension is a science - based diet to lower high blood pressure. It is one of the most effective science-based diets for reducing high blood pressure.

The DASH diet is mainly based on fruits, vegetables, whole grains, legumes, nuts, seeds and low-fat dairy products. It is promoted by adding fruits and vegetables, as well as nuts and seeds, such as almonds, avocados, walnuts, peaches, oranges, cherries, pears, grapes, apples, bananas, strawberries, tomatoes, cucumbers, etc.

Before you start a diet or any other diet, talk to a doctor about the health benefits of different types of foods such as fruits, vegetables, whole grains, legumes, nuts, seeds, etc.

It is important to remember that the DASH diet is a healthy lifestyle that can help lower blood pressure. If you want to lose weight with a dash diet, you probably need to reduce calories. Whether you are a dietitian or want to adjust your diet, here is everything you need to know about the best foods for high blood pressure., 17

In summary, the DASH diet allows you to eat delicious, healthy meals with lots of vegetables, various fruits and good protein sources. Here is a quick cookbook on how to add a little salt to create your own dash diet plan with ease.

Nutritional approaches to control hypertension, based on two studies that looked at the reduction of blood pressure during dietary changes.

Participants who ate the DASH diet and consumed less sodium had lower blood pressure, and the results showed that there was no difference in the combined effect of the two diets in terms of blood pressure. A reduction in sodium through the "DASH" diet can lower blood pressure: "The results show that a diet with additional fruits and vegetables lowers blood pressure compared to the first diet. If the reduced sodium intake is accompanied by a dash diet, the diet with lower sodium content is promoted. The results show that there is a positive correlation between a diet rich in sodium, high in fruit and vegetables and a lower risk of hypertension.

The DASH diet also includes fish, poultry and legumes and promotes small amounts of nuts and seeds several times a week. The main study examined the dash diet and there were two randomized diets, with one control diet mirroring the typical American diet and resembling the standard diet of a typical healthy adult in the United States. They provided a list of fruits, vegetables and whole grains recommended for the "DASH" diet, as well as a description of the diet.

Although the two diets are similar, the DASH diet has more precise guidelines and was originally developed to treat hypertension. Most doctors and dieticians recommend the original plan for patients with high blood pressure. While Americans limit their daily sodium intake to less than 2,300 mg per day, you can meet the standard for the "DASH" diet by consuming 1,500 milligrams of sodium per day on the low-sodium diet plan. You can also eat up to 1 million mg of protein and 1.5 million grams of carbohydrates per week on a "low-sodium" diet plan, and 2.2 million mg / day on an "average" "normal" "dash diet.

Research on the DASH diet supports the idea that your eating habits can improve certain health markers, including blood pressure and total cholesterol. Although the original research was long ago, scientists are conducting a meta-analysis of the "DASH" diet to see how much it can lower blood pressure. In this study, a high-fat version, which includes a high-protein, low-carbohydrate diet, and a low-sodium version, were compared to a dash diet, and both successfully lowered blood pressure in the study.

BREAKFAST

1. Quinoa Hashes

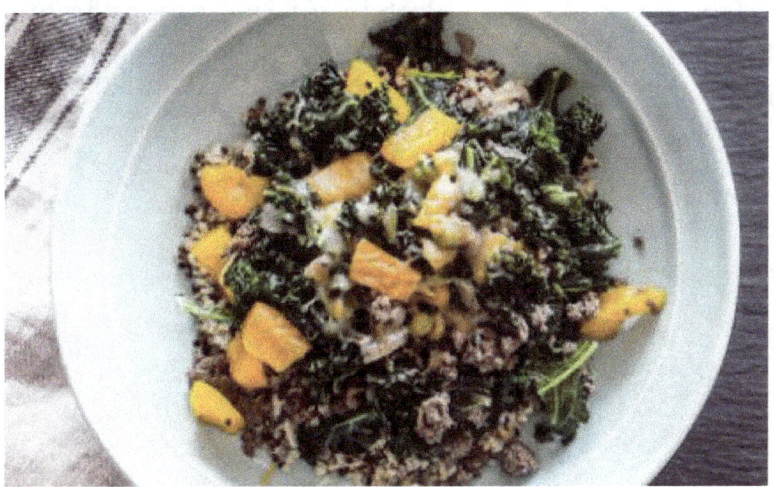

Preparation time: 10 minutes

Cooking time: 25 minutes

Servings: 2

Ingredients:

- 3 oz. quinoa
- 6 oz. water
- 2 potatoes, grated
- 1 egg, beaten
- 1 tablespoon avocado oil
- 1 teaspoon chives, chopped

Directions:

1. Cook quinoa in water for 15 minutes.
2. Heat up avocado oil in the skillet.

3. Then mix up all remaining ingredients in the bowl. Add quinoa and mix up well.

4. Add quinoa hash browns, cook for 5 minutes on each side.

Nutrition: 344 Calories, 12.5g Protein, 61.3g Carbohydrates, 5.9g Fat, 8.4g Fiber, 82mg Cholesterol, 49mg Sodium, 1160mg Potassium.

2.Artichoke Eggs

Preparation time: 5 minutes

Cooking time: 20 minutes

Servings: 4

Ingredients:

- 5 eggs, beaten
- 2 oz. low-fat feta, chopped
- 1 yellow onion, chopped
- 1 tablespoon canola oil
- 1 tablespoon cilantro, chopped
- 1 cup artichoke hearts, canned, chopped

Directions:

1. Grease 4 ramekins with the oil.
2. Mix up all remaining ingredients and divide the mixture between prepared ramekins.
3. Bake the meal at 380F for 20 minutes.

Nutrition: 177 Calories, 10.6 Protein, 7.4g Carbohydrates, 12.2g Fat, 2.5g Fiber, 217mg Cholesterol, 259mg Sodium, 235mg Potassium.

3.Quinoa Cakes

Preparation time: 25 minutes

Cooking time: 10 minutes

Servings: 4

Ingredients:

- 7 oz. quinoa
- 1 cup cauliflower, shredded
- 1 cup of water
- ½ cup vegan parmesan, grated
- 1 egg, beaten
- 1 tablespoon olive oil
- ½ teaspoon ground black pepper

Directions:

1. Mix up the quinoa with the cauliflower, water, and ground black pepper, stir, bring to a simmer over medium heat and cook for 15 minutes/
2. Cool the mixture and add parmesan and the eggs, stir well, shape medium cakes out of this mix.
3. Heat up a pan with the oil over medium-high heat, add the quinoa cakes. Cook them for 4-5 minutes per side.

Nutrition: 280 Calories, 14.9g Protein, 36.4g Carbohydrates, 7.6g Fat, 4.2g Fiber, 41mg Cholesterol, 222mg Sodium, 374mg Potassium.

4. Bean Casserole

Preparation time: 10 minutes

Cooking time: 30 minutes

Servings: 8

Ingredients:

- 5 eggs, beaten
- ½ cup bell pepper, chopped
- 1 cup red kidney beans, cooked
- ½ cup white onions, chopped
- 1 cup low-fat mozzarella cheese, shredded

Directions:

1. Spread the beans over the casserole mold. Add onions and bell pepper.
2. Add the eggs mixed with the cheese.
3. Bake the casserole 380 F for 30 minutes.

Nutrition: 142 Calories, 12.8g Protein, 16g Carbohydrates, 3g Fat, 4.3g Fiber, 105mg Cholesterol, 162mg Sodium, 374mg Potassium.

5.Grape Yogurt

Preparation time: 10 minutes

Cooking time: 0 minutes

Servings: 3

Ingredients:

- 1 ½ cup low-fat yogurt
- ½ cup grapes, chopped
- 1 oz. walnuts, chopped

Directions:

1. Mix up all ingredients together and transfer them in the serving glasses.

Nutrition:

156 Calories, 9.4g Protein, 12.2g Carbohydrates, 7.1g Fat, 0.8g Fiber, 7mg Cholesterol, 86mg Sodium, 365mg Potassium.

LUNCH

6.Pasta Primavera

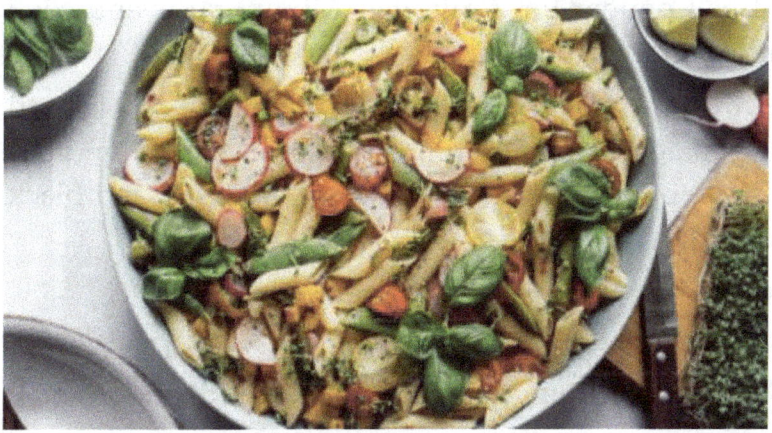

Preparation time: 10 minutes

Cooking time: 25 minutes

Servings: 4

Ingredients:

- 2 cups cauliflower florets, cut into matchsticks
- 16 oz. tortiglioni
- ¼ cup olive oil
- ½ cup chopped fresh green onions
- 1 red bell pepper, thinly sliced
- 4 garlic cloves, minced
- 1 cup grape tomatoes, halved
- 2 tsp. dried Italian seasoning
- ½ lemon, juiced
- ½ cup grated Pecorino Romano cheese

Directions:

1. In a pot of boiling water, cook the tortiglioni pasta for 8-10 minutes until al dente. Drain and set aside.

2. Heat olive oil in a skillet and sauté onion, cauliflower, and bell pepper for 7 minutes. Mix in garlic and cook until fragrant, 30 seconds.

3. Stir in the tomatoes and Italian seasoning; cook until the tomatoes soften, 5 minutes. Mix in the lemon juice and tortiglioni and adjust the taste with salt and black pepper.

4. Garnish with the Pecorino Romano cheese.

Nutrition: Calories: 381; Protein: 25.3 Grams; Fat: 12.9 Grams; Carbs: 9.7 Grams; Sodium: 480 mg; Cholesterol: 37 mg

7.Delicious Chicken Pasta

Preparation Time: 10 minutes

Cooking Time: 17 minutes

Servings: 4

Ingredients:

- 3 chicken breasts, skinless, boneless, cut into pieces
- 9 oz. whole-grain pasta
- 1/2 cup olives, sliced
- 1/2 cup sun-dried tomatoes
- 1 tbsp. roasted red peppers, chopped
- 14 oz. can tomatoes, diced
- 2 cups marinara sauce
- 1 cup chicken broth
- Pepper
- Salt

Directions:

1. Add all ingredients except whole-grain pasta into the instant pot and stir well. Seal pot with lid and cook on high for 12 minutes.

2. Once done, allow to release pressure naturally. Remove lid. Add pasta and stir well. Seal pot again and select manual and set timer for 5 minutes.

3. Once done, allow to release pressure naturally for 5 minutes then release remaining using quick release. Remove lid. Stir well and serve.

Nutrition: Calories: 381; Protein: 25.3 Grams; Fat: 12.9 Grams; Carbs: 9.7 Grams; Sodium: 480 mg; Cholesterol: 37 mg

8.Flavorful Mac & Cheese

Preparation Time: 10 minutes

Cooking Time: 10 minutes

Servings: 6

Ingredients:

- 16 oz. whole-grain elbow pasta
- 4 cups of water
- 1 cup can tomatoes, diced
- 1 tsp. garlic, chopped
- 2 tbsp. olive oil
- 1/4 cup green onions, chopped
- 1/2 cup parmesan cheese, grated
- 1/2 cup mozzarella cheese, grated
- 1 cup cheddar cheese, grated
- 1/4 cup passata
- 1 cup unsweetened almond milk
- 1 cup marinated artichoke, diced
- 1/2 cup sun-dried tomatoes, sliced
- 1/2 cup olives, sliced
- 1 tsp. salt

Directions

1. Add pasta, water, tomatoes, garlic, oil, and salt into the instant pot and stir well. Seal pot with lid and cook on high for 4 minutes.

2. Once done, allow to release pressure naturally for 5 minutes then release remaining using quick release. Remove lid. Set pot on sauté mode.

3. Add green onion, parmesan cheese, mozzarella cheese, cheddar cheese, passata, almond milk, artichoke, sun-dried tomatoes, and olive. Mix well. Stir well and cook until cheese is melted. Serve and enjoy.

Nutrition: Calories: 381; Protein: 25.3 Grams; Fat: 12.9 Grams; Carbs: 9.7 Grams; Sodium: 480 mg; Cholesterol: 37 mg

9.Flavors Herb Risotto

Preparation Time: 10 minutes

Cooking Time: 15 minutes

Servings: 4

Ingredients:

- 2 cups of rice
- 2 tbsp. parmesan cheese, grated
- oz. heavy cream
- 1 tbsp. fresh oregano, chopped
- 1 tbsp. fresh basil, chopped
- 1/2 tbsp. sage, chopped
- 1 onion, chopped
- 2 tbsp. olive oil
- 1 tsp. garlic, minced
- 4 cups vegetable stock
- Pepper
- Salt

Directions:

1. Add oil into the inner pot of instant pot and set the pot on sauté mode. Add garlic and onion and sauté for 2-3 minutes.
2. Add remaining ingredients except for parmesan cheese and heavy cream and stir well. Seal pot with lid and cook on high for 12 minutes.

3. Once done, allow to release pressure naturally for 10 minutes then release remaining using quick release. Remove lid. Stir in cream and cheese and serve.

Nutrition: Calories: 381; Protein: 25.3 Grams; Fat: 12.9 Grams; Carbs: 9.7 Grams; Sodium: 480 mg; Cholesterol: 37 mg

10.Delicious Pasta Primavera

Preparation Time: 10 minutes

Cooking Time: 4 minutes

Servings: 4

Ingredients:

- 8 oz. whole wheat penne pasta
- 1 tbsp. fresh lemon juice
- 2 tbsp. fresh parsley, chopped
- 1/4 cup almonds slivered
- 1/4 cup parmesan cheese, grated
- 14 oz. can tomatoes, diced
- 1/2 cup prunes
- 1/2 cup zucchini, chopped
- 1/2 cup asparagus, cut into 1-inch pieces
- 1/2 cup carrots, chopped
- 1/2 cup broccoli, chopped
- 1 3/4 cups vegetable stock
- Pepper
- Salt

Directions:

1. Add stock, pars, tomatoes, prunes, zucchini, asparagus, carrots, and broccoli into the instant pot and stir well. Seal pot with lid and cook on high for 4 minutes.

2. Once done, release pressure using quick release. Remove lid. Add remaining ingredients and stir well and serve.

Nutrition: Calories: 381; Protein: 25.3 Grams; Fat: 12.9 Grams; Carbs: 9.7 Grams; Sodium: 480 mg; Cholesterol: 37 mg

DINNER

The Almond Breaded Chicken Goodness

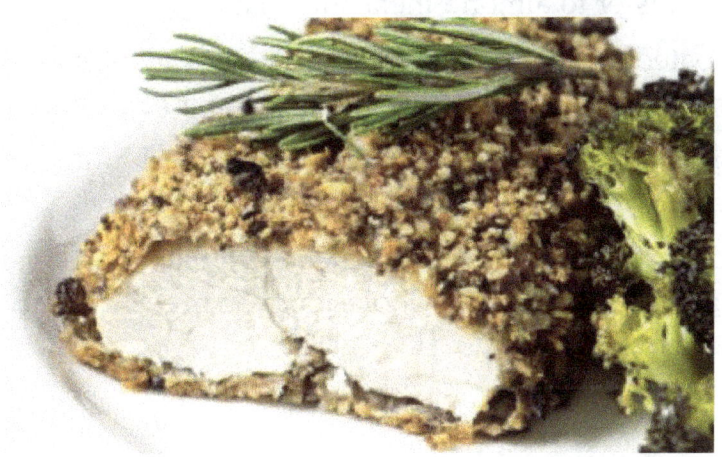

Preparation Time: 15 minutes

Cooking Time: 15 minutes

Servings: 3

Ingredients:

- 2 large chicken breasts, boneless and skinless
- 1/3 cup lemon juice
- 1 ½ cups seasoned almond meal
- 2 tablespoons coconut oil
- Lemon pepper, to taste
- Parsley for decoration

Directions:

1. Slice chicken breast in half. Pound out each half until ¼ inch thick.

2. Take a pan and place it over medium heat, add oil and heat it up. Dip each chicken breast slice into lemon juice and let it sit for 2 minutes.

3. Turnover and the let the other side sit for 2 minutes as well. Transfer to almond meal and coat both sides.

4. Add coated chicken to the oil and fry for 4 minutes per side, making sure to sprinkle lemon pepper liberally.

5. Transfer to a paper lined sheet and repeat until all chicken are fried. Garnish with parsley and enjoy!

Nutrition: Calories: 128; Protein: 21 Grams; Fat: 4 Grams; Carbs: 3 Grams; Sodium: 81 mg; Cholesterol: 55 mg

Almond butter Pork Chops

Preparation Time: 5 minutes

Cooking Time: 25 minutes

Servings: 3

Ingredients:

- 1 tablespoon almond butter, divided
- 2 boneless pork chops
- Pepper to taste
- 1 tablespoon dried Italian seasoning, low fat and low sodium
- 1 tablespoon olive oil

Directions:

1. Pre-heat your oven to 350 degrees F. Pat pork chops dry with a paper towel and place them in a baking dish.

2. Season with pepper, and Italian seasoning. Drizzle olive oil over pork chops. Top each chop with ½ tablespoon almond butter.

3. Bake for 25 minutes. Transfer pork chops on two plates and top with almond butter juice. Serve and enjoy!

Nutrition: Calories: 128; Protein: 21 Grams; Fat: 4 Grams; Carbs: 3 Grams; Sodium: 81 mg; Cholesterol: 55 mg

Healthy Mediterranean Lamb Chops

Preparation Time: 10 minutes

Cooking Time: 10 minute

Servings: 2

Ingredients:

- 4 lamb shoulder chops,
- 8 ounces each
- 2 tablespoons Dijon mustard
- 2 tablespoons Balsamic vinegar
- ½ cup olive oil
- 2 tablespoons shredded fresh basil

Directions:

1. Pat your lamb chop dry using a kitchen towel and arrange them on a shallow glass baking dish. Take a bowl and a whisk in Dijon mustard, balsamic vinegar, pepper and mix them well.

2. Whisk in the oil very slowly into the marinade until the mixture is smooth Stir in basil. Pour the marinade over the lamb chops and stir to coat both sides well.

3. Cover the chops and allow them to marinate for 1-4 hours (chilled). Take the chops out and leave them for 30 minutes to allow the temperature to reach a normal level.

4. Pre-heat your grill to medium heat and add oil to the grate. Grill the lamb chops for 5-10 minutes per side until both sides are browned. Once the center reads 145 degrees F, the chops are ready, serve and enjoy!

Nutrition: Calories: 128; Protein: 21 Grams; Fat: 4 Grams; Carbs: 3 Grams; Sodium: 81 mg; Cholesterol: 55 mg

Brown Butter Duck Breast

Preparation Time: 5 minutes

Cooking Time: 25 minutes

Servings: 3

Ingredients:

- 1 whole 6 ounce duck breast, skin on
- Pepper to taste
- 1 head radicchio
- 4 ounces, core removed
- ¼ cup unsalted butter
- 6 fresh sage leaves, sliced

Directions:

1. Pre-heat your oven to 400 degree F. Pat duck breast dry with paper towel. Season with pepper.
2. Place duck breast in skillet and place it over medium heat, sear for 3-4 minutes each side. Turn breast over and transfer skillet to oven.
3. Roast for 10 minutes (uncovered). Cut radicchio in half. Remove and discard the woody white core and thinly slice the leaves. Keep them on the side.
4. Remove skillet from oven. Transfer duck breast, fat side up to cutting board and let it rest. Re-heat your skillet over medium heat.
5. Add unsalted butter, sage and cook for 3-4 minutes. Cut duck into 6 equal slices. Divide radicchio between 2 plates, top with slices of duck breast and drizzle browned butter and sage. Enjoy!

Nutrition: Calories: 128; Protein: 21 Grams; Fat: 4 Grams; Carbs: 3 Grams; Sodium: 81 mg; Cholesterol: 55 mg

Chipotle Lettuce Chicken

Preparation Time: 10 minutes

Cooking Time: 25 minutes

Servings: 6

Ingredients:

- 1 pound chicken breast, cut into strips
- Splash of olive oil
- 1 red onion, finely sliced
- 14 ounces tomatoes
- 1 teaspoon chipotle, chopped
- ½ teaspoon cumin
- Lettuce as needed
- Fresh coriander leaves
- Jalapeno chilies, sliced
- Fresh tomato slices for garnish
- Lime wedges

Directions:

1. Take a non-stick frying pan and place it over medium heat. Add oil and heat it up.

2. Add chicken and cook until brown. Keep the chicken on the side.

3. Add tomatoes, sugar, chipotle, cumin to the same pan and simmer for 25 minutes until you have a nice sauce. Add chicken into the sauce and cook for 5 minutes.

4. Transfer the mix to another place. Use lettuce wraps to take a portion of the mixture and serve with a squeeze of lemon. Enjoy!

Nutrition: Calories: 128; Protein: 21 Grams; Fat: 4 Grams; Carbs: 3 Grams; Sodium: 81 mg; Cholesterol: 55 mg

MAINS

Cauliflower Tabbouleh

Preparation time: 10 minutes

Cooking time: 4 minutes

Servings: 4

Ingredients:

- 1-pound cauliflower head
- 1 cucumber, chopped
- 2 tablespoons lemon juice
- 2 tablespoons olive oil
- ½ cup fresh parsley
- 1 garlic clove, diced
- 1 oz. scallions, chopped
- 1 teaspoon mint

Directions:

1. Trim and chop cauliflower head. Transfer it in the food processor and pulse until you get cauliflower rice.

2. Transfer the cauliflower rice in the glass mixing bowl. Add lemon juice and chopped scallions. Mix up the mixture.

3. Microwave it for 4 minutes.

4. Meanwhile, blend together olive oil, parsley, and diced garlic.

5. Mix up together cooked cauliflower rice with parsley mixture. Add mint and chopped cucumbers.

6. Mix it up and transfer on the serving plates.

Nutrition: Calories 108, Fat 7.3, Fiber 3.7, Carbs 10.2, Protein 3.2

Stuffed Artichoke

Preparation time: 10 minutes

Cooking time: 15 minutes

Servings: 4

Ingredients:

- 2 artichokes
- 4 tablespoon Parmesan, grated
- 2 teaspoon almond flour
- 1 teaspoon minced garlic
- 3 tablespoons sour cream
- 1 teaspoon avocado oil
- 1 cup water, for cooking

Directions:

1. Pour water in the saucepan and bring it to boil.
2. When the water is boiling, add artichokes and boil them for 5 minutes.
3. Drain water from artichokes and trim them.
4. Remove the artichoke hearts.
5. Preheat the oven to 365F.
6. Mix up together almond flour, grated Parmesan, minced garlic, sour cream, and avocado oil.
7. Fill the artichokes with cheese mixture and place on the baking tray.
8. Cook the vegetables for 10 minutes.
9. Then cut every artichoke into halves and transfer on the serving plates.

Nutrition: Calories 162, Fat 10.7, Fiber 5.9, Carbs 12.4, Protein 8.2

Beef Salpicao

Preparation time: 10 minutes

Cooking time: 18 minutes

Servings: 2

Ingredients:

- 1-pound rib eye, boneless
- 2 garlic cloves, peeled, diced
- 2 tablespoons butter
- 1 tablespoon sour cream
- ½ teaspoon salt
- ½ teaspoon chili pepper
- 1 tablespoon lime juice

Directions:

1. Cut rib eye into the strips.
2. Sprinkle the meat with salt, chili pepper, and lime juice.
3. Toss butter in the skillet. Add diced garlic and roast it for 2 minutes over the medium heat.
4. Then add meat strips and roast them over the high heat for 2 minutes from each side.
5. Add sour cream and close the lid. Cook the meal for 10 minutes more over the medium heat. Stir it from time to time.
6. Transfer cooked beef Salpicao on the serving plates.

Nutrition: Calories 641, Fat 52.8, Fiber 0.1, Carbs 1.9, Protein 42.5

Cream Dredged Corn Platter

Preparation Time: 10 minutes

Cooking Time: 4 hours

Servings: 3

Ingredients:

- 3 cups corn
- 2 ounces cream cheese, cubed
- 2 tablespoons milk
- 2 tablespoons whipping cream
- 2 tablespoons butter, melted
- Salt and pepper as needed
- 1 tablespoon green onion, chopped

Directions:

1. Add corn, cream cheese, milk, whipping cream, butter, salt and pepper to your Slow Cooker.
2. Give it a nice toss to mix everything well. Place lid and cook on LOW for 4 hours.
3. Divide the mix amongst serving platters. Serve and enjoy!

Nutrition: Calories 641, Fat 52.8, Fiber 0.1, Carbs 1.9, Protein 42.5

Ethiopian Cabbage Delight

Preparation Time: 15 minutes

Cooking Time: 6- 8 hours

Servings: 6

Ingredients:

- ½ cup water
- 1 head green cabbage, cored and chopped
- 1 pound sweet potatoes, peeled and chopped
- 3 carrots, peeled and chopped
- 1 onion, sliced
- 1 teaspoon extra virgin olive oil
- ½ teaspoon ground turmeric
- ½ teaspoon ground cumin
- ¼ teaspoon ground ginger

Directions:

1. Add water to your Slow Cooker. Take a medium bowl and add cabbage, carrots, sweet potatoes, onion and mix.
2. Add olive oil, turmeric, ginger, cumin and toss until the veggies are fully coated.
3. Transfer veggie mix to your Slow Cooker. Cover and cook on LOW for 6-8 hours. Serve and enjoy!

Nutrition: Calories 641, Fat 52.8, Fiber 0.1, Carbs 1.9, Protein 42.5

SIDES AND APPETIZERS

Mediterranean Pop Corn Bites

Preparation time: 5 minutes + 20 minutes chill

Cooking time: 2-3 minutes

Servings: 4

Ingredients:

- 3 cups Medjool dates, chopped
- 12 ounces brewed coffee
- cup pecan, chopped
- ½ cup coconut, shredded
- ½ cup cocoa powder

Directions:

1. Soak dates in warm coffee for 5 minutes.
2. Remove dates from coffee and mash them, making a fine smooth mixture.
3. Stir in remaining ingredients (except cocoa powder) and form small balls out of the mixture.
4. Coat with cocoa powder, serve and enjoy!

Nutrition: Calories: 265; Fat: 12g; Carbohydrates: 43g; Protein 3g

Hearty Buttery Walnuts

Preparation time: 10 minutes

Cooking time: 20 minutes

Servings: 4

Ingredients:

- 4 walnut halves
- ½ tablespoon almond butter

Directions:

1. Spread butter over two walnut halves.
2. Top with other halves.
3. Serve and enjoy!

Nutrition: Calories: 90; Fat: 10g; Carbohydrates: 0g; Protein: 1g

Refreshing Watermelon Sorbet

Preparation time: 20 minutes + 20 hours chill time

Cooking time: 20 minutes

Servings: 4

Ingredients:

- 4 cups watermelon, seedless and chunked
- ¼ cup coconut sugar
- 2 tablespoons lime juice

Directions:

1. Add the listed ingredients to a blender and puree.
2. Transfer to a freezer container with a tight-fitting lid.
3. Freeze the mix for about 4-6 hours until you have gelatin-like consistency.
4. Puree the mix once again in batches and return to the container.
5. Chill overnight.
6. Allow the sorbet to stand for 5 minutes before serving and enjoy!

Nutrition: Calories: 91; Fat: 0g; Carbohydrates: 25g; Protein: 1g

Lovely Faux Mac and Cheese

Preparation time: 15 minutes

Cooking time: 45 minutes

Servings: 4

Ingredients:

- 5 cups cauliflower florets
- Salt and pepper to taste
- cup coconut milk
- ½ cup vegetable broth
- tablespoons coconut flour, sifted
- organic egg, beaten
- cups cheddar cheese

Directions:

1. Pre-heat your oven to 350 degrees F.
2. Season florets with salt and steam until firm.
3. Place florets in greased ovenproof dish.
4. Heat coconut milk over medium heat in a skillet, make sure to season the oil with salt and pepper.
5. Stir in broth and add coconut flour to the mix, stir.
6. Cook until the sauce begins to bubble.
7. Remove heat and add beaten egg.
8. Pour the thick sauce over cauliflower and mix in cheese.
9. Bake for 30-45 minutes.
10. Serve and enjoy!

Nutrition: Calories: 229; Fat: 14g; Carbohydrates: 9g; Protein: 15g

Beautiful Banana Custard

Preparation time: 10 minutes

Cooking time: 25 minutes

Servings: 3

Ingredients:

- 2 ripe bananas, peeled and mashed finely
- ½ teaspoon of vanilla extract
- 14-ounce unsweetened almond milk
- 3 eggs

Directions:

1. Pre-heat your oven to 350 degrees F.
2. Grease 8 custard glasses lightly.
3. Arrange the glasses in a large baking dish.
4. Take a large bowl and mix all of the ingredients and mix them well until combined nicely.
5. Divide the mixture evenly between the glasses.
6. Pour water in the baking dish.
7. Bake for 25 minutes.
8. Take out and serve.
9. Enjoy!

Nutrition: Calories: 59; Fat: 2.4g; Carbohydrates: 7g; Protein: 3g

SEAFOOD

Lemon Garlic Shrimp

Preparation time: 15 minutes

Cooking time: 10 minutes

Servings: 4

Ingredients:

- 2 tablespoons extra-virgin olive oil
- 3 garlic cloves, sliced
- ½ teaspoon kosher salt
- ¼ teaspoon red pepper flakes
- 1-pound large shrimp, peeled and deveined
- ½ cup white wine
- 3 tablespoons fresh parsley, minced
- Zest of ½ lemon
- Juice of ½ lemon

Directions:

1. Heat-up the olive oil in a wok or large skillet over medium-high heat. Add the garlic, salt, and red pepper flakes and sauté until the garlic starts to brown, 30 seconds to 1 minute.

2. Add the shrimp and cook within 2 to 3 minutes on each side. Pour in the wine and deglaze the wok, scraping up any flavorful brown bits, for 1 to 2 minutes. Turn off the heat; mix in the parsley, lemon zest, and lemon juice.

Nutrition: Calories: 200; Fat: 9g; Sodium: 310mg; Carbohydrates: 3g; Protein: 23g

Shrimp Fra Diavolo

Preparation time: 15 minutes

Cooking time: 10 minutes

Servings: 4

Ingredients:

- 2 tablespoons extra-virgin olive oil
- onion, diced small
- 1 fennel bulb, cored and diced small, plus ¼ cup fronds for garnish
- 1 bell pepper, diced small
- ½ teaspoon dried oregano
- ½ teaspoon dried thyme
- ½ teaspoon kosher salt
- ¼ teaspoon red pepper flakes
- 1 (14.5-ounce) can no-salt-added diced tomatoes
- 1-pound shrimp, peeled and deveined
- Juice of 1 lemon
- Zest of 1 lemon
- tablespoons fresh parsley, chopped, for garnish

Directions:

1. Heat-up the olive oil in a large skillet or sauté pan over medium heat. Add the onion, fennel, bell pepper, oregano, thyme, salt, and red pepper flakes and sauté until translucent, about 5 minutes.

2. Drizzle the pan using the canned tomatoes' juice, scraping up any brown bits, and bringing to a boil. Add

the diced tomatoes and the shrimp. Lower heat to a simmer within 3 minutes.

3. Turn off the heat. Add the lemon juice and lemon zest, and toss well to combine. Garnish with the parsley and the fennel fronds.

Nutrition: Calories: 240; Fat: 9g; Sodium: 335mg; Carbohydrates: 13g; Protein: 25g

Fish Amandine

Preparation time: 15 minutes

Cooking time: 15 minutes

Servings: 4

Ingredients:

- 4-ounce skinless tilapia, trout, or halibut fillets, 1/2- to 1-inch thick
- ¼ cup buttermilk
- ½ teaspoon dry mustard
- 1/8 teaspoon crushed red pepper
- tablespoon butter, melted
- ¼ teaspoon salt
- ½ cup panko bread crumbs
- tbsp. chopped fresh parsley
- ¼ cup sliced almonds, coarsely chopped
- tablespoons grated Parmesan cheese

Directions:

1. Defrost fish, if frozen. Preheat oven to 450oF. Grease a shallow baking pan; set aside. Rinse fish; pat dry with paper towels.

2. Pour buttermilk into a shallow dish. In an extra shallow dish, mix bread crumbs, dry mustard, parsley, and salt. Soak fish into buttermilk, then into crumb mixture, turning to coat. Put coated fish in the ready baking pan.

3. Flavor the fish with almonds plus Parmesan cheese; drizzle with melted butter. Sprinkle with crinkled red

pepper. Bake for 5 minutes per 1/2-inch thickness of fish or until fish flakes easily when checked with a fork.

Nutrition: Calories 209; Fat 8.7 g; Sodium 302 mg; Carbohydrates 6.7 g; Protein 26.2 g

Air-Fryer Fish Cakes

Preparation time: 15 minutes

Cooking time: 10 minutes

Servings: 2

Ingredients:

- Cooking spray
- 10 oz. finely chopped white fish
- 2/3 cup whole-wheat panko breadcrumbs
- 3 tablespoons finely chopped fresh Cilantro
- 2 tablespoons Thai sweet chili sauce
- 2 tablespoons canola mayonnaise
- large egg
- 1/8 teaspoon salt
- ¼ teaspoon ground pepper
- lime wedges

Directions:

1. Oiled the basket of an air fryer with cooking spray. Put fish, cilantro, panko, chili sauce, egg, mayonnaise, pepper, and salt in a medium bowl; stir until well mixed. Shape the mixture into four 3-inch-diameter cakes.

2. Oiled the cakes with cooking spray; place in the basket. Cook at 400oF until the cakes are browned for 9 to 10 minutes. Serve with lime wedges.

Nutrition: Calories 399; Fat 15.5 g; Sodium 537 mg; Carbohydrates 27.9 g; Protein 34.6 g

Pesto Shrimp Pasta

Preparation time: 15 minutes

Cooking time: 12 minutes

Servings: 4

Ingredients:

- 1/8 teaspoon freshly cracked pepper
- cup dried orzo
- 4 tsp. packaged pesto sauce mix
- 1 lemon, halved
- 1/8 teaspoon coarse salt
- 1-pound medium shrimp, thawed
- 1 medium zucchini, halved lengthwise and sliced
- tablespoons olive oil, divided
- 1-ounce shaved Parmesan cheese

Directions:

1. Prepare orzo pasta concerning package directions. Drain; reserving ¼ cup of the pasta cooking water. Mix 1 teaspoon of the pesto mix into the kept cooking water and set aside.

2. Mix 3 teaspoons of the pesto mix plus 1 tablespoon of the olive oil in a large plastic bag. Seal and shake to mix. Put the shrimp in the bag; seal and turn to coat. Set aside.

3. Sauté zucchini in a big skillet over moderate heat for 1 to 2 minutes, stirring repeatedly. Put the pesto-marinated shrimp in the skillet and cook for 5 minutes or until shrimp is dense.

4. Put the cooked pasta in the skillet with the zucchini and shrimp combination. Stir in the kept pasta water until absorbed, grating up any seasoning in the bottom of the pan. Season with pepper and salt. Squeeze the lemon over the pasta. Top with Parmesan, then serve.

Nutrition: Calories 361; Fat 10.1 g; Sodium 502 mg; Carbohydrates 35.8 g; Protein 31.6 g

POULTRY

Chicken Sliders

Preparation time: 10 minutes

Cooking time: 10 minutes

Servings: 4

Ingredients:

- 10 ounces ground chicken breast
- 1 tablespoon black pepper
- 1 tablespoon minced garlic
- 1 tablespoon balsamic vinegar
- 1/2 cup minced onion
- 1 fresh chili pepper, minced
- 1 tablespoon fennel seed, crushed
- 4 whole-wheat mini buns
- 4 lettuce leaves
- 4 tomato slices

Directions:

1. Combine all the ingredients except the wheat buns, tomato, and lettuce. Mix well and refrigerate the mixture for 1 hour. Divide the mixture into 4 patties.

2. Broil these patties in a greased baking tray until golden brown. Place the chicken patties in the wheat buns along with lettuce and tomato. Serve.

Nutrition: Calories 224; Fat 4.5 g; Sodium 212 mg; Carbs 10.2 g; Protein 67.4 g

White Chicken Chili

Preparation time: 20 minutes

Cooking time: 15 minutes

Servings: 4

Ingredients:

- 1 can white chunk chicken
- 2 cans low-sodium white beans, drained
- 1 can low-sodium diced tomatoes
- 4 cups of low-sodium chicken broth
- 1 medium onion, chopped
- 1/2 medium green pepper, chopped
- 1 medium red pepper, chopped
- 2 garlic cloves, minced
- 2 teaspoons chili powder
- 1 teaspoon ground cumin
- 1 teaspoon dried oregano
- Cayenne pepper, to taste
- 8 tablespoons shredded reduced-fat Monterey Jack cheese
- 3 tablespoons chopped fresh cilantro

Directions:

1. In a soup pot, add beans, tomatoes, chicken, and chicken broth. Cover this soup pot and let it simmer over medium heat. Meanwhile, grease a nonstick pan with cooking spray. Add peppers, garlic, and onions. Sauté for 5 minutes until soft.

2. Transfer the mixture to the soup pot. Add cumin, chili powder, cayenne pepper, and oregano. Cook for 10 minutes, then garnish the chili with cilantro and 1 tablespoon cheese. Serve.

Nutrition: Calories 225; Fat 12.9 g; Sodium 480 mg; Carbs 24.7 g; Protein 25.3g

Sweet Potato-Turkey Meatloaf

Preparation time: 15 minutes

Cooking time: 25 minutes

Servings: 4

Ingredients:

- 1 large sweet potato, peeled and cubed
- 1-pound ground turkey (breast)
- 1 large egg
- 1 small sweet onion, finely chopped
- 2 cloves garlic, minced
- 2 slices whole-wheat bread, crumbs
- ¼ cup honey barbecue sauce
- ¼ cup ketchup
- 2 Tablespoons Dijon Mustard
- 1 Tablespoon fresh ground pepper
- ½ Tablespoon salt

Directions:

1. Warm oven to 350 F. Grease a baking dish. In a large pot, boil a cup of lightly salted water, add the sweet potato. Cook until tender. Drain the water. Mash the potato.

2. Mix the honey barbecue sauce, ketchup, and Dijon mustard in a small bowl. Mix thoroughly. In a large bowl, mix the turkey and the egg. Add the sweet onion, garlic. Pour in the combined sauces. Add the bread crumbs. Season the mixture with salt and pepper.

3. Add the sweet potato. Combine thoroughly with your hands. If the mixture feels wet, add more bread crumbs. Shape the mixture into a loaf. Place in the loaf pan. Bake for 25 – 35 minutes until the meat is cooked through. Broil for 5 minutes. Slice and serve.

Nutrition: Calories – 133; Protein - 85g; Carbohydrates - 50g; Fat - 34g; Sodium - 202mg

Oaxacan Chicken

Preparation time: 15 minutes

Cooking time: 28 minutes

Servings: 2

Ingredients:

- 1 4-ounce chicken breast, skinned and halved
- ½ cup uncooked long-grain rice
- 1 teaspoon of extra-virgin olive oil
- ½ cup low-sodium salsa
- ½ cup chicken stock, mixed with 2 Tablespoons water
- ¾ cup baby carrots
- 2 tablespoons green olives, pitted and chopped
- 2 Tablespoons dark raisins
- ½ teaspoon ground Cinnamon
- 2 Tablespoons fresh cilantro or parsley, coarsely chopped

Directions:

1. Warm oven to 350 F. In a large saucepan that can go in the oven, heat the olive oil. Add the rice. Sauté the rice until it begins to pop, approximately 2 minutes.

2. Add the salsa, baby carrots, green olives, dark raisins, halved chicken breast, chicken stock, and ground cinnamon. Bring the mix to a simmer, stir once.

3. Cover the mixture tightly, bake in the oven until the chicken stock has been completely absorbed, approximately 25 minutes. Sprinkle fresh cilantro or parsley, mix. Serve immediately.

Nutrition: Calories – 143; Protein - 102g; Carbohydrates - 66g. Fat - 18g. Sodium - 97mg

Spicy Chicken with Minty Couscous

Preparation time: 15 minutes

Cooking time: 25 minutes

Servings: 2

Ingredients:

- 2 small chicken breasts, sliced
- 1 red chili pepper, finely chopped
- 1 garlic clove, crushed
- ginger root, 2 cm long peeled and grated
- 1 teaspoon ground cumin
- ½ teaspoon turmeric
- 2 Tablespoons extra-virgin olive oil
- 1 pinch sea salt
- ¾ cup couscous
- Small bunch mint leaves, finely chopped
- 2 lemons, grate the rind and juice them

Directions:

1. In a large bowl, place the chicken breast slices and chopped chili pepper. Sprinkle with the crushed garlic, ginger, cumin, turmeric, and a pinch of salt. Add the grated rind of both lemons and the juice from 1 lemon. Pour 1 tablespoon of the olive oil over the chicken, coat evenly.

2. Cover the dish with plastic and refrigerate within 1 hour. After 1 hour, coat a skillet with olive oil and fry the chicken. As the chicken is cooking, pour the

couscous into a bowl and pour hot water over it, let it absorb the water (approximately 5 minutes).

3. Fluff the couscous. Add some chopped mint, the other tablespoon of olive oil, and juice from the second lemon. Top the couscous with the chicken. Garnish with chopped mint. Serve immediately.

Nutrition: Calories – 166; Protein - 106g; Carbohydrates - 52g; Sugars - 0.1g; Fat - 17g; Sodium - 108mg

Chicken, Pasta and Snow Peas

Preparation time: 15 minutes

Cooking time: 20 minutes

Servings: 2

Ingredients:

- 1-pound chicken breasts
- 2 ½ cups penne pasta
- 1 cup snow peas, trimmed and halved
- 1 teaspoon olive oil
- 1 standard jar Tomato and Basil pasta sauce
- Fresh ground pepper

Directions:

1. In a medium frying pan, heat the olive oil. Flavor the chicken breasts with salt and pepper. Cook the chicken breasts until cooked through (approximately 5 – 7 minutes each side).

2. Cook the pasta, as stated in the instruction of the package. Cook the snow peas with the pasta. Scoop 1 cup of the pasta water. Drain the pasta and peas, set aside.

3. Once the chicken is cooked, slice diagonally. Return back the chicken in the frying pan. Add the pasta sauce. If the mixture seems dry, add some of the pasta water to the desired consistency. Heat, then divide into bowls. Serve immediately.

Nutrition: Calories – 140; Protein - 34g; Carbohydrates - 52g; Fat - 17g; Sodium - 118mg

Chicken with Noodles

Preparation time: 15 minutes

Cooking time: 30 minutes

Servings: 6

Ingredients:

- 4 chicken breasts, skinless, boneless
- 1-pound pasta (angel hair, or linguine, or ramen)
- ½ teaspoon sesame oil
- 1 Tablespoon canola oil
- 2 Tablespoons chili paste
- 1 onion, diced
- 2 garlic cloves, chopped coarsely
- ½ cup of soy sauce
- ½ medium cabbage, sliced
- 2 carrots, chopped coarsely

Directions:

1. Cook your pasta in a large pot. Mix the canola oil, sesame oil, and chili paste and heat for 25 seconds in a large pot. Add the onion, cook for 2 minutes. Put the garlic and fry within 20 seconds. Add the chicken, cook on each side 5 - 7 minutes, until cooked through.

2. Remove the mix from the pan, set aside. Add the cabbage, carrots, cook until the vegetables are tender. Pour everything back into the pan. Add the noodles. Pour in the soy sauce and combine thoroughly. Heat for 5 minutes. Serve immediately.

Nutrition: Calories – 110; Protein - 30g; Carbohydrates - 32g; Sugars - 0.1g; Fat - 18g; Sodium - 121mg

MEAT

Pork Tenderloin with Apples and Balsamic Vinegar

Preparation time: 10 Minutes

Cooking Time: 25 minutes

Servings: 4

Ingredients:

- 1 tablespoon olive oil
- 1-pound pork tenderloin, trimmed from fat
- Freshly ground black pepper
- 2 cups chopped onion
- 2 cups chopped apple
- 1 ½ tablespoons fresh rosemary, chopped
- 1 cup low sodium chicken broth
- 1 ½ tablespoons balsamic vinegar

Directions:

1. Heat the oven to 4500F.
2. Heat the oil in a large skillet over medium flame.
3. Sear the pork and season with black pepper. Cook the pork for 3 minutes until all sides turn light brown. Remove from the heat and place in a baking pan.
4. Roast the pork for 15 minutes.
5. Meanwhile, place the onion, apples, and rosemary on the skillet where the pork is seared. Continue stirring

for 5 minutes. Pour in broth and balsamic vinegar and allow to simmer until the sauce thickens.

6. Serve the roasted pork with the onion and apple sauce.

Nutrition: Calories: 240; Protein: 26g; Carbs: 17g; Fat: 6g; Saturated Fat: 1g; Sodium: 83mg

Pork Tenderloin with Apples and Blue Cheese

Preparation time: 10 Minutes

Cooking Time: 25 minutes

Servings: 4

Ingredients:

- 1-pound pork tenderloin, trimmed from fat
- ½ teaspoon white pepper
- 2 teaspoons black pepper
- ¼ teaspoon cayenne pepper
- 1 teaspoon paprika
- 2 apples, sliced
- ½ cup unsweetened apple juice
- ¼ cup crumbled blue cheese

Directions:

1. Heat the oven to 3500F.
2. Season the tenderloin with white pepper, black pepper, cayenne pepper, and paprika.
3. Heat a non-stick pan over medium flame and sear the meat for 3 minutes on each side. Transfer to a baking dish and roast in the oven for 20 minutes or until the internal temperature is at 1550F. Remove from the oven to cool.
4. While the pork is roasting, prepare the sauce. Using the same skillet used to sear the meat, sauté the apples for 3 minutes. Add the apple juice and allow the sauce to thicken for at least 10 minutes.

5. Serve the pork with the apple sauce and sprinkle with blue cheese on top.

Nutrition: Calories: 235; Protein: 26g; Carbs: 17; Fat: 3g; Saturated Fat: 1g; Sodium: 145mg

Pork Tenderloin with Fennel Sauce

Preparation time: 10 Minutes

Cooking Time: 30 minutes

Servings: 4

Ingredients:

- 4 pork tenderloin fillets, trimmed from fat and cut into 4 portions
- 1 tablespoon olive oil
- 1 teaspoon fennel seeds
- 1 fennel bulb, cored and sliced thinly
- 1 sweet onion, sliced thinly
- ½ cup dry white wine
- 12 ounces low sodium chicken broth
- 1 orange, sliced for garnish

Directions:

1. Place the pork slices in between wax paper and pound with a mallet to about ¼-inch thick.

2. Heat oil in a skillet and fry the fennel seeds for 3 minutes or until fragrant.

3. Stir in the pork and cook on all sides for 3 minutes or until golden brown. Remove the pork from the skillet and set aside.

4. Using the same skillet, add the fennel bulb slices and onion. Sauté for 5 minutes then set aside.

5. Add the wine and chicken broth in the skillet and bring to a boil until the sauce reduces in half.

6. Return the pork to the skillet and cook for another 5 minutes.

7. Serve the pork with sauce and vegetables.

Nutrition: Calories: 276; Protein: 29g; Carbs: 13g; Fat: 12g; Saturated Fat: 3 g; Sodium: 122mg

Spicy Beef Kebabs

Preparation time: 10 Minutes

Cooking Time: 10 minutes

Servings: 8

Ingredients:

- 2 yellow onions, minced
- 2 tablespoons fresh lemon juice
- 1 ½ pounds lean ground beef, minced
- ¼ cup bulgur, soaked in water for 30 minutes then rinsed
- ¼ cup chopped pine nuts
- 2 cloves of garlic, minced
- 1 teaspoon ground cumin
- ½ teaspoon ground cinnamon
- ½ teaspoon ground cardamom
- ½ teaspoon freshly ground black pepper
- 16 wooden skewers, soaked in water for 30 minutes

Directions:

1. In a mixing bowl, combine all ingredients except for the skewers. Mix well unto

2. Form a sausage from the meat mixture and thread it into the skewers. If the sausage is crumbly, add a tablespoon of water at a time until it holds well together. Refrigerate the skewered meat sausages until ready to cook.

3. Heat the grill to 3500F and place the grill rack 6 inches from the heat source.

4. Place the skewered kebabs on the grill and broil for 5 minutes on each side.

5. Serve with yogurt if desired.

Nutrition: Calories: 219; Protein: 23g; Carbs: 3g; Fat: 12g; Saturated Fat: 3g; Sodium: 53mg

Spicy Beef Curry

Preparation time: 10 Minutes

Cooking Time: 40 minutes

Servings: 6

Ingredients:

- 1 medium serrano pepper, cut into thirds
- 4 cloves of garlic, minced
- 1 2-inch piece ginger, peeled and chopped
- 1 yellow onion, chopped
- 2 tablespoon ground coriander
- 2 teaspoons ground cumin
- ½ teaspoon ground turmeric
- 2 teaspoons garam masala
- 1 tablespoon olive oil
- pounds beef, cut into chunks
- 1 cup ripe tomatoes, diced
- 2 cups water
- 1 cup fresh cilantro for garnish

Directions:

1. In a food processor, pulse the serrano peppers, garlic, ginger, onion, coriander, cumin, turmeric, and garam masala until well-combined.

2. Heat oil over medium heat in a skillet and sauté the spice mixture for 2 minutes or until fragrant.

3. Stir in the beef and allow to cook while stirring constantly for three minutes or until the beef turns brown.

4. Stir in the tomatoes and sauté for another three minutes.

5. Add in the water and bring to a boil.

6. Once boiling, turn the heat to low and allow to simmer for thirty minutes or until the meat is tender.

7. Add cilantro last before serving.

Nutrition: Calories: 181; Protein: 16g; Carbs: 5g; Fat: 8g; Saturated Fat: 2g; Sodium: 74mg

Pork Tenderloin with Apples and Sweet Potatoes

Preparation time: 10 Minutes

Cooking Time: 30 minutes

Servings: 4

Ingredients:

- ¾ cup apple cider
- ¼ cup apple cider vinegar
- 2 tablespoons maple syrup
- ¼ teaspoon smoked paprika powder
- 1 teaspoon grated ginger
- ¼ teaspoon ground black pepper
- 2 teaspoons olive oil
- 1 12-ounce pork tenderloin
- 1 large sweet potato, cut into cubes
- 1 large apple, cored and into cubes

Directions:

1. Preheat the oven to 3750F.

2. In a bowl, combine the apple cider, apple cider vinegar, maple syrup, smoked paprika, ginger, and black pepper. Set aside.

3. Heat the oil in a large skillet and sear the meat for 3 minutes on both sides.

4. Transfer the pork in a baking dish and place the sweet potatoes and apples around the pork. Pour in the apple cider sauce.

5. Place inside the oven and cook for 20 minutes.

Nutrition: Calories: 267; Protein: 23.5g; Carbs: 31 g; Fat: 5g; Saturated Fat: 0.5g; Sodium: 69mg

VEGETABLES

Loaded Baked Sweet Potatoes

Preparation time: 15 minutes

Cooking time: 20 minutes

Servings: 4

Ingredients:

- 4 sweet potatoes
- ½ cup nonfat or low-fat plain Greek yogurt
- Freshly ground black pepper
- 1 teaspoon olive oil
- 1 red bell pepper, cored and diced
- ½ red onion, diced
- 1 teaspoon ground cumin
- 1 (15-ounce) can chickpeas, drained and rinsed

Directions:

1. Prick the potatoes using a fork and cook on your microwave's potato setting until potatoes are soft and cooked through, about 8 to 10 minutes for 4 potatoes. If you don't have a microwave, bake at 400°F for about 45 minutes.

2. Combine the yogurt and black pepper in a small bowl and mix well. Heat the oil in a medium pot over medium heat. Add bell pepper, onion, cumin, and additional black pepper to taste.

3. Add the chickpeas, stir to combine, and heat through about 5 minutes. Slice the potatoes lengthwise down the middle and top each half with a portion of the bean mixture followed by 1 to 2 tablespoons of the yogurt. Serve immediately.

Nutrition: Calories: 264 Fat: 2g Sodium: 124mg Carbohydrate: 51g Protein: 11g

White Beans with Spinach and Pan-Roasted Tomatoes

Preparation time: 15 minutes

Cooking time: 10 minutes

Servings: 2

Ingredients:

- 1 tablespoon olive oil
- 4 small plum tomatoes, halved lengthwise
- 10 ounces frozen spinach, defrosted and squeezed of excess water
- 2 garlic cloves, thinly sliced
- 2 tablespoons water
- ¼ teaspoon freshly ground black pepper
- 1 can white beans, drained
- Juice of 1 lemon

Directions:

1. Heat-up the oil in a large skillet over medium-high heat. Put the tomatoes, cut-side down, and cook within 3 to 5 minutes; turn and cook within 1 minute more. Transfer to a plate.

2. Reduce heat to medium and add the spinach, garlic, water, and pepper to the skillet. Cook, tossing until the spinach is heated through, 2 to 3 minutes.

3. Return the tomatoes to the skillet, put the white beans and lemon juice, and toss until heated through 1 to 2 minutes.

Nutrition: Calories: 293 Fat: 9g Sodium: 267mg Carbohydrate: 43g Protein: 15g

Black-Eyed Peas and Greens Power Salad

Preparation time: 15 minutes

Cooking time: 6 minutes Servings: 2

Ingredients:

- 1 tablespoon olive oil
- 3 cups purple cabbage, chopped
- 5 cups baby spinach
- 1 cup shredded carrots
- 1 can black-eyed peas, drained
- Juice of ½ lemon
- Salt
- Freshly ground black pepper

Directions:

1. In a medium pan, add the oil and cabbage and sauté for 1 to 2 minutes on medium heat. Add in your spinach, cover for 3 to 4 minutes on medium heat, until greens are wilted. Remove from the heat and add to a large bowl.

2. Add in the carrots, black-eyed peas, and a splash of lemon juice. Season with salt and pepper, if desired. Toss and serve.

Nutrition: Calories: 320 Fat: 9g Sodium: 351mg Potassium: 544mg Carbohydrate: 49g Protein: 16g

Butternut-Squash Macaroni and Cheese

Preparation time: 15 minutes

Cooking time: 20 minutes

Servings: 2

Ingredients:

- 1 cup whole-wheat ziti macaroni
- 2 cups peeled and cubed butternut squash
- 1 cup nonfat or low-fat milk, divided
- Freshly ground black pepper
- 1 teaspoon Dijon mustard
- 1 tablespoon olive oil
- ¼ cup shredded low-fat cheddar cheese

Directions:

1. Cook the pasta al dente. Put the butternut squash plus ½ cup milk in a medium saucepan and place over medium-high heat. Season with black pepper. Bring it to a simmer. Lower the heat, then cook until fork-tender, 8 to 10 minutes.

2. To a blender, add squash and Dijon mustard. Purée until smooth. Meanwhile, place a large sauté pan over medium heat and add olive oil. Add the squash purée and the remaining ½ cup of milk. Simmer within 5 minutes. Add the cheese and stir to combine.

3. Add the pasta to the sauté pan and stir to combine. Serve immediately.

Nutrition: Calories: 373 Fat: 10g Sodium: 193mg Carbohydrate: 59g Protein: 14g

Pasta with Tomatoes and Peas

Preparation time: 15 minutes

Cooking time: 15 minutes

Servings: 2

Ingredients:

- ½ cup whole-grain pasta of choice
- 8 cups water, plus ¼ for finishing
- 1 cup frozen peas
- 1 tablespoon olive oil
- 1 cup cherry tomatoes, halved
- ¼ teaspoon freshly ground black pepper
- 1 teaspoon dried basil
- ¼ cup grated Parmesan cheese (low-sodium)

Directions:

1. Cook the pasta al dente. Add the water to the same pot you used to cook the pasta, and when it's boiling, add the peas. Cook within 5 minutes. Drain and set aside.

2. Heat-up the oil in a large skillet over medium heat. Add the cherry tomatoes, put a lid on the skillet and let the tomatoes soften for about 5 minutes, stirring a few times.

3. Season with black pepper and basil. Toss in the pasta, peas, and ¼ cup of water, stir and remove from the heat. Serve topped with Parmesan.

Nutrition: Calories: 266 Fat: 12g Sodium: 320mg Carbohydrate: 30g Protein: 13g

SNACKS AND DESSERTS

The Mean Green Smoothie

Preparation time: 5 minutes

Cooking time: 10 minutes

Serving: 2

Ingredients:

- 1 avocado
- 1 handful spinach, chopped
- Cucumber, 2 inch slices, peeled
- 1 lime, chopped
- Handful of grapes, chopped
- 5 dates, stoned and chopped
- 1 cup apple juice (fresh)

Directions:

1. Add all the listed ingredients to your blender.
2. Blend until smooth.
3. Add a few ice cubes and serve the smoothie.
4. Enjoy!

Nutrition: Calories: 200; Fat: 10g; Carbohydrates: 14g; Protein 2g

Mint Flavored Pear Smoothie

Preparation time: 5 minutes

Cooking time: 5 minutes

Serving: 2

Ingredients:

- ¼ honey dew
- 2 green pears, ripe
- ½ apple, juiced
- 1 cup ice cubes
- ½ cup fresh mint leaves

Directions:

1. Add the listed ingredients to your blender and blend until smooth.
2. Serve chilled!

Nutrition: Calories: 200; Fat: 10g; Carbohydrates: 14g; Protein 2g

Chilled Watermelon Smoothie

Preparation time: 5 minutes

Cooking time: 10 minutes

Serving: 2

Ingredients:

- 1 cup watermelon chunks
- ½ cup coconut water
- 1 ½ teaspoons lime juice
- 4 mint leaves
- 4 ice cubes

Directions:

1. Add the listed ingredients to your blender and blend until smooth.
2. Serve chilled!

Nutrition: Calories: 200; Fat: 10g; Carbohydrates: 14g; Protein 2g

Banana Ginger Medley

Preparation time: 5 minutes

Cooking time: 10 minutes

Serving: 2

Ingredients:

- 1 banana, sliced
- ¾ cup vanilla yogurt
- 1 tablespoon honey
- ½ teaspoon ginger, grated

Directions:

1. Add the listed ingredients to your blender and blend until smooth.
2. Serve chilled!

Nutrition: Calories: 200; Fat: 10g; Carbohydrates: 14g; Protein 2g

Banana and Almond Flax Glass

Preparation time: 5 minutes

Cooking time: 10 minutes

Serving: 2

Ingredients:

- 1 ripe frozen banana, diced
- 2/3 cup unsweetened almond milk
- 1/3 cup fat free plain Greek Yogurt
- 1 ½ tablespoons almond butter
- 1 tablespoon flaxseed meal
- 1 teaspoon honey
- 2-3 drops almond extract

Directions:

1. Add the listed ingredients to your blender and blend until smooth
2. Serve chilled!

Nutrition: Calories: 200; Fat: 10g; Carbohydrates: 14g; Protein 2g

Sensational Strawberry Medley

Preparation time: 5 minutes

Cooking time: 10 minutes

Serving: 2

Ingredients:

- 1-2 handful baby greens
- 3 medium kale leaves
- 5-8 mint leaves
- 1 inch piece ginger , peeled
- 1 avocado
- 1 cup strawberries
- 6-8 ounces coconut water + 6-8 ounces filtered water
- Fresh juice of one lime
- 1-2 teaspoon olive oil

Directions:

1. Add all the listed ingredients to your blender.
2. Blend until smooth.
3. Add a few ice cubes and serve the smoothie.
4. Enjoy!

Nutrition: Calories: 200; Fat: 10g; Carbohydrates: 14g; Protein 2g

Sweet Almond and Coconut Fat Bombs

Preparation time: 10 minutes

Cooking Time: /Freeze Time: 20 minutes

Serving: 6

Ingredients:

- ¼ cup melted coconut oil
- 9 ½ tablespoons almond butter
- 90 drops liquid stevia
- 3 tablespoons cocoa
- 9 tablespoons melted butter, salted

Directions:

1. Take a bowl and add all of the listed ingredients.
2. Mix them well.
3. Pour scant 2 tablespoons of the mixture into as many muffin molds as you like.
4. Chill for 20 minutes and pop them out.
5. Serve and enjoy!

Nutrition: Total Carbs: 2g; Fiber: 0g; Protein: 2.53g; Fat: 14g

Almond and Tomato Balls

Preparation time: 10 minutes

Cooking Time: Freeze Time: 20 minutes

Servings: 6

Ingredients:

- 1/3 cup pistachios, de-shelled
- 10 ounces cream cheese
- 1/3 cup sun dried tomatoes, diced

Directions:

1. Chop pistachios into small pieces.
2. Add cream cheese, tomatoes in a bowl and mix well.
3. Chill for 15-20 minutes and turn into balls.
4. Roll into pistachios.
5. Serve and enjoy!

Nutrition: Carb: 183; Fat: 18g; Carb: 5g; Protein: 5g

Avocado Tuna Bites

Preparation time: 10 minutes

Cooking Time: Nil

Serving: 4

Ingredients:

1/3 cup coconut oil

1 avocado, cut into cubes

10 ounces canned tuna, drained

¼ cup parmesan cheese, grated

¼ teaspoon garlic powder

1/4 teaspoon onion powder

1/3 cup almond flour

¼ teaspoon pepper

¼ cup low fat mayonnaise

Pepper as needed

Directions:

Take a bowl and add tuna, mayo, flour, parmesan, spices and mix well.

Fold in avocado and make 12 balls out of the mixture.

Melt coconut oil in pan and cook over medium heat, until all sides are golden.

Serve and enjoy!

Nutrition: Calories: 185; Fat: 18g; Carbohydrates: 1g; Protein: 5g

Mediterranean Pop Corn Bites

Preparation time: 5 minutes + 20 minutes chill time

Cooking Time: 2-3 minutes

Servings: 4

Ingredients:

3 cups Medjool dates, chopped

12 ounces brewed coffee

1 cup pecan, chopped

½ cup coconut, shredded

½ cup cocoa powder

Directions:

Soak dates in warm coffee for 5 minutes.

Remove dates from coffee and mash them, making a fine smooth mixture.

Stir in remaining ingredients (except cocoa powder) and form small balls out of the mixture.

Coat with cocoa powder, serve and enjoy!

Nutrition: Calories: 265; Fat: 12g; Carbohydrates: 43g; Protein 3g

Hearty Buttery Walnuts

Preparation time: 10 minutes

Cooking Time: Nil

Serving: 4

Ingredients:

4 walnut halves

½ tablespoon almond butter

Directions:

Spread butter over two walnut halves.

Top with other halves.

Serve and enjoy!

Nutrition: Calories: 90; Fat: 10g; Carbohydrates: 0g; Protein: 1g

Refreshing Watermelon Sorbet

Preparation time: 20 minutes + 20 hours chill time

Cooking Time: Nil

Serving: 4

Ingredients:

4 cups watermelon, seedless and chunked

¼ cup coconut sugar

2 tablespoons lime juice

Directions:

Add the listed ingredients to a blender and puree.

Transfer to a freezer container with a tight-fitting lid.

Freeze the mix for about 4-6 hours until you have gelatin-like consistency.

Puree the mix once again in batches and return to the container.

Chill overnight.

Allow the sorbet to stand for 5 minutes before serving and enjoy!

Nutrition: Calories: 91; Fat: 0g; Carbohydrates: 25g; Protein: 1g

CPSIA information can be obtained
at www.ICGtesting.com
Printed in the USA
BVHW091947180521
607636BV00010B/1406